SELF HEAL BY DESIGN DIET COOKBOOK

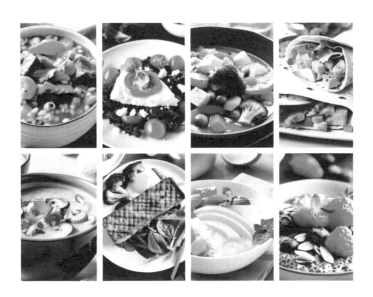

The Ultimate Health Guide With Delicious and Nourishing Recipes to Balance Your Micro-organisms

CULINARY CHRONICLES

Copyright © 2023 by Culinary Chronicles

All rights reserved. No part of this publication may be reproduced, distributed, or transmitted in any form or by any means, including photocopying, recording, or other electronic or mechanical methods, without the prior written permission of the publisher, except in the case of brief quotations embodied in critical reviews and certain other noncommercial uses permitted by copyright law.

The information provided in this book is intended for informational purposes only and should not be construed as professional or expert advice. Readers should consult with appropriate professionals before making any decisions or taking any actions based on the content of this book. The author and publisher disclaim any liability or responsibility for any losses or damages that may result, directly or indirectly, from the use of the information in this book.

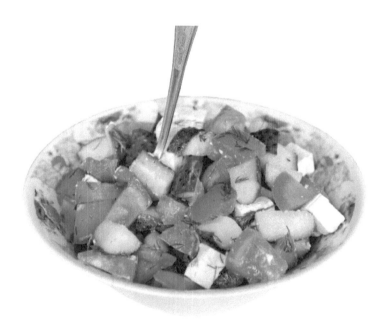

TABLE OF CONTENTS

Introduction (6)
Chapter 1: The Power of Nutrition: A Journey to Healing (8)
Understanding the Body's Natural Healing Process (11)
The Role of Microorganisms in Our Diet (14)

Chapter 2: Foundations of Healing Nutrition (17)
The Basic Principles of a Healing Diet (17)
Essential Nutrients for Optimal Health (20)
The Gut Microbiome: Our Internal Ecosystem (22)

Chapter 3: Energising Breakfast Bowls (25)
Quinoa Berry Bliss Bowl (25)
Tropical Mango & Coconut Bowl (26)
Chia Seed Power Bowl (27)
Savory Veggie & Hummus Bowl (28)
Nutty Avocado Bowl (29)
Mediterranean Breakfast Bowl (30)
Tempeh & Greens Breakfast Bowl (31)
Seeded Greek Yogurt Bowl (32)
Hearty Chickpea Salad Bowl (33)
Nuts & Berries Greek Yogurt Bowl (34)

Chapter 4: Nourishing Porridges & Overnight Oats (35)
Golden Turmeric Porridge (35)
Creamy Coconut & Chia Porridge (36)
Cinnamon Apple Porridge (37)
Classic Berry Overnight Oats (38)
Tropical Mango & Coconut Overnight Oats (39)
Peanut Butter & Banana Overnight Oats (40)
Chocolate Almond Overnight Oats (41)
Mixed Berry and Chia Seed Porridge (42)
Golden Turmeric Overnight Oats (43)
Creamy Coconut and Date Porridge (44)

Chapter 5: Revitalising Smoothies & Juices (45)
Green Powerhouse Smoothie (45)
Berry Bliss Smoothie (45)
Tropical Turmeric Smoothie (46)
Peanut Butter & Banana Smoothie (47)
Chocolate Almond Smoothie (47)
Refreshing Green Juice (48)
Sunrise Citrus Juice (49)
Beetroot Boost Juice (49)
Zesty Ginger Tonic (50)

Chapter 6: Wholesome Salads (51)
Quinoa & Roasted Veggie Salad (51)
Kale & Avocado Bliss Salad (52)
Chickpea & Spinach Power Salad (53)
Roasted Beet & Goat Cheese Salad (54)
Mediterranean Tuna Salad (55)
Broccoli & Toasted Almond Salad (56)
Thai Inspired Mango Salad (57)
Cabbage & Sesame Seed Crunch Salad (58)
Sun-Dried Tomato & Spinach Pasta Salad (59)
Greek Inspired Chickpea Salad (60)

Chapter 7: Healing Soups and Stews (61)
Nourishing Bone Broth Soup (61)
Creamy Lentil & Spinach Soup (62)
Healing Turmeric & Ginger Soup (63)
Immunity-Boosting Mushroom Soup (64)
Wholesome Vegetable Stew (65)
Rejuvenating Beet Soup (Borscht) (66)
Heart-Warming Pumpkin Soup (67)
Revitalising Fish Stew (68)

Chapter 8: Plant-Powered Main Courses (70)
Stuffed Bell Peppers with Quinoa & Veggies (70)
Eggplant & Chickpea Curry (71)
Lentil & Vegetable Shepherd's Pie (72)
Zucchini Noodle Stir-Fry with Tofu (73)
Cauliflower Steak with Pesto (74)
Chickpea & Spinach Curry (75)
Vegan Eggplant Parmesan (76)
Vegan Lentil Loaf (77)
Vegan Risotto with Asparagus & Mushrooms (78)
Vegan Stuffed Acorn Squash (79)

Chapter 9: Comforting One-Pot Dinner Meals (80)
Tuscan White Bean & Kale Stew (80)
One-Pot Vegetable & Chickpea Curry (81)
One-Pot Vegan Chili (82)
One-Pot Lentil & Mushroom Stroganoff (83)
Mediterranean One-Pot Orzo & Veggies (84)
Vegan Spanish Paella (85)
Creamy Vegan One-Pot Pasta (86)
One-Pot Moroccan Chickpea Tagine (87)
One-Pot Vegan Jambalaya (88)
Vegan Potato & Leek Soup (89)

Chapter 10: 28-Day Meal Plan (90)

Chapter 11: Crafting a Year-Long Meal Journey: A Blueprint for Wholesome Living (98)

Chapter 12: 1500 Days of Recipes: Mastering the Art of Culinary Variation (101)

Conclusion: Nourishing Your Way to Wellness (104)

Bonus: Meal Planning Journal (105)

Introduction

In every corner of the world, from bustling metropolises to tranquil villages, food stands as a universal language. It carries tales of culture, love, tradition, and survival. But beyond its rich tapestry of flavours and memories, food possesses an even more profound capability—it has the potential to heal.

Welcome to the "Self Heal by Design Diet Cookbook." Within these pages, you embark on a culinary journey where every bite, every ingredient, and every recipe is meticulously chosen, not just for its delightful taste, but for its restorative powers. This is not just a collection of recipes; it's a guide to reconnecting with the very essence of our beings, understanding that our bodies, when provided the right nourishment, can manifest miracles.

Since time immemorial, our ancestors believed in the remedial properties of certain foods. They didn't have the luxury of modern medicine, so they turned to nature, to the roots, herbs, and berries that grew in their backyards. They cooked with intention, understanding that every meal was an opportunity to bolster the body's defences, to soothe ailments, and to nurture the soul.

Modern science now confirms what ancient wisdom has long professed: the gut is our second brain. The microorganisms thriving within play an instrumental role in not just our physical well-being, but our mental and emotional states as well. Our diets, in essence, have the power to shape our moods, our vitality, and our overall health.

So, what does it mean to 'self heal by design'? It's a commitment, a conscious choice to embrace foods that nourish and fortify. It's about recognizing the signals our bodies send us, acknowledging the innate wisdom they hold, and providing them the sustenance they crave to repair, rejuvenate, and thrive.

This cookbook is designed to be your companion in this exploration, offering recipes that are as delectable as they are beneficial.

Whether you're a seasoned chef or a kitchen novice, the recipes herein invite you to explore, experiment, and enjoy. More than just satiating hunger, they're crafted to serve your body's deeper needs, balancing your internal ecosystem, and harnessing the therapeutic wonders of ingredients.

As you turn the pages and dive into these recipes, remember that each dish is an act of self-love, a step towards a life where healing isn't sought but is designed by you, for you. Embrace this journey, relish every bite, and let your body's natural ability to self heal unfold deliciously.

Chapter 1: The Power of Nutrition: A Journey to Healing

In the mosaic of life, where we seek purpose, happiness, and well-being, there's one element that we often overlook: the profound power of nutrition. This power doesn't just refer to the ability of food to satiate our hunger or tantalise your taste buds. It's about the intrinsic relationship between what we consume and our body's capacity to heal, regenerate, and thrive.

The Science Behind Nutritional Healing

Every morsel of food that we ingest undergoes a complex journey of transformation. Carbohydrates are broken down into sugars that fuel our cells, proteins into amino acids that repair our tissues, and fats into fatty acids that support cellular structure and function. Beyond these basic nutrients, our foods are packed with vitamins, minerals, and phytochemicals that play critical roles in countless physiological processes.

Research has shown how certain nutrients can expedite wound healing, how others can enhance immune response, and still others can influence mood and cognitive function. For instance, omega-3 fatty acids, found in fatty fish and flaxseeds, have anti-inflammatory properties and can reduce the risk of chronic diseases. Similarly, antioxidants like vitamin C and E combat oxidative stress, which can otherwise accelerate ageing and heighten disease risk.

Listening to Our Bodies

The journey to healing through nutrition starts by tuning into our bodies. The body, in its infinite wisdom, often signals its needs, deficiencies, or excesses. That persistent fatigue might be an iron deficiency, while those recurrent mood swings could be linked to an imbalance in blood sugar levels or essential fatty acids.

Nutrition as Preventive Medicine

While modern medicine excels in treating symptoms and acute conditions, nutrition offers a proactive approach, preventing ailments before they manifest. By providing our bodies with a balanced spectrum of nutrients, we bolster our defence mechanisms, reduce inflammation, and ensure optimal function of all organ systems.

Gut Health: The Epicentre of Well-being

The gut isn't just a digestive organ; it's a hub of immunity, mood regulation, and even hormone production. With an intricate ecosystem of microorganisms, our gut health is integral to overall well-being. Foods rich in probiotics and prebiotics—like yoghourt, kimchi, and whole grains—foster a healthy microbiome, further underscoring the symbiotic relationship between nutrition and health.

Tailoring Nutrition for Healing

There's no one-size-fits-all when it comes to nutrition. Our genetic makeup, lifestyle, age, and specific health challenges all influence our nutritional requirements. By understanding these variables, we can tailor a diet that not only promotes healing but also resonates with our personal needs and preferences.

Conclusion

The path to healing isn't a straight line; it's a journey filled with discovery, learning, and adaptation. Through the lens of nutrition, we're equipped with a potent tool—one that empowers us to influence our health's trajectory actively. In the tapestry of life's experiences, our choices at the dining table weave a narrative of resilience, healing, and holistic well-being. In recognizing and harnessing the power of nutrition, we embark on one of the most transformative journeys—a journey to healing.

Understanding the Body's Natural Healing Process

In the intricate dance of life, our bodies constantly face challenges—be it environmental toxins, pathogens, injuries, or emotional stress. However, evolution has bestowed us with an intricate healing mechanism, a system so sophisticated that it often works seamlessly without our conscious intervention. To truly harness our body's potential for self-healing, as highlighted, we must first understand this incredible process.

The Innate Immune Response

When faced with an immediate threat, such as a wound or bacterial invasion, the body's innate immune response kicks into gear. This is a generalised defence mechanism, which includes barriers like our skin, mucosal linings, and the acid in our stomach. White blood cells, such as neutrophils and macrophages, are dispatched to the site of injury or infection, where they work to engulf pathogens and remove debris.

The Adaptive Immune Response

While the innate immune response acts rapidly, the adaptive immune system takes a more tailored approach. It detects specific pathogens and remembers them for any future encounters. Lymphocytes, which include T-cells and B-cells, play a crucial role here. When they encounter a recognized invader, they proliferate and mount a targeted defence, producing antibodies that neutralise the threat.

Inflammation: A Double-edged Sword

Inflammation refers to the body's natural response to injury or infection. It serves to isolate the affected area, prevent the spread of pathogens, and facilitate healing. Symptoms include redness, heat, swelling, and sometimes pain. While acute inflammation is beneficial and vital, chronic inflammation, often stemming from lifestyle factors like poor diet or stress, can be detrimental and underlie many chronic diseases.

Cellular Repair and Regeneration

Our bodies are designed to be in a constant state of turnover. Cells undergo wear and tear, DNA experiences damage, and tissues can be injured. However, many of our cells have the capacity to divide and regenerate. Stem cells in particular, found in various parts of the body, can differentiate into diverse cell types, aiding in tissue repair. Moreover, mechanisms like autophagy help clean out damaged cells, allowing for the generation of healthier ones.

The Role of Nutrition and Environment

Nutrition plays an invaluable role in supporting the body's healing processes. Vitamins like C and E have antioxidant properties that combat cellular damage. Minerals like zinc and magnesium facilitate DNA repair and immune function. Omega-3 fatty acids modulate inflammation. Moreover, external factors like clean air, sunlight (vitamin D synthesis), and sleep quality profoundly influence our healing capabilities.

Emotional and Mental Well-being

Physical health doesn't exist in isolation. Our emotional and mental states significantly influence our body's ability to heal. Chronic stress, for instance, can suppress the immune response, while positive emotions and mindfulness practices can enhance our healing capacity.

Conclusion

The body's natural healing process is a testament to the marvels of evolution. It's a sophisticated orchestra of responses, finely tuned and interlinked. By understanding this mechanism, as elucidated in "Self Heal by Design," we are better equipped to support and facilitate our inherent healing journey. Through conscious lifestyle choices, nutrition, mental well-being, and respecting our body's signals, we can truly optimise our health and well-being.

The Role of Microorganisms in Our Diet

Amidst the vast tapestry of the human body's workings, a surprising but crucial player emerges: micro-organisms. Our body is a teeming ecosystem, home to trillions of microbes that coexist with us, playing an instrumental role in our health and well-being. These microscopic entities, primarily found in our gut but also on our skin and other orifices, have a profound influence on various physiological processes. Their significance becomes even more pronounced when we consider the impact of our diet on this microbial community.

The Human Microbiome: A Brief Overview

Our body hosts a complex consortium of bacteria, viruses, fungi, and other microorganisms collectively referred to as the microbiome. The largest concentration of this microbiome resides in our gut, particularly the large intestine. These microbes have evolved with us over millennia, engaging in a symbiotic relationship where both parties benefit.

Digestion and Nutrient Absorption

One of the primary roles of gut bacteria is aiding in digestion. Some fibres and complex carbohydrates cannot be broken down by our digestive enzymes. Gut bacteria metabolise these substances, producing short-chain fatty acids (SCFAs) in the process. SCFAs, such as butyrate, propionate, and acetate, are pivotal for colon health, providing energy to colon cells and possessing anti-inflammatory properties.

Immune System Modulation

The gut is a major immunological site. Gut microbes play a crucial role in educating and modulating our immune system. A balanced microbiome ensures an optimal immune response—vigorous enough to combat pathogens but regulated to prevent excessive inflammation or autoimmune reactions.

Mood and Neurotransmitter Production

Emerging research suggests a gut-brain axis, where gut microbes influence brain function and behaviour. Certain gut bacteria produce neurotransmitters, such as serotonin and dopamine. Additionally, the gut microbiome can influence inflammation and other factors that have implications for mental health.

Dietary Impact on the Microbiome

Our dietary choices exert a profound impact on the composition and function of our gut microbiome. A diet rich in diverse plant-based foods fosters a varied microbiome, which is often associated with health benefits. On the contrary, diets high in processed foods, sugars, and unhealthy fats can lead to a less diverse microbial community, potentially increasing disease risk.
Fermented foods, like yoghourt, sauerkraut, and kimchi, introduce beneficial bacteria into our gut. Prebiotic foods, such as onions, garlic, and whole grains, provide the necessary fibers and nutrients to nourish these microbes.

Microbes Beyond the Gut

While the gut microbiome receives much attention, it's crucial to recognize that beneficial microbes are also present in foods that influence other parts of our body. For instance, fermented dairy or skin products can influence the skin's microbiome, impacting skin health.

Conclusion

The intricate dance between our body and its resident microorganisms is a testament to nature's complexity and interconnectedness. Recognizing the role of these microbes and nurturing them through optimal dietary choices is pivotal for holistic health. By doing so, we harness the power of an invisible army, working tirelessly to ensure our well-being from the inside out.

Chapter 2: Foundations of Healing Nutrition

The Basic Principles of a Healing Diet

The journey to holistic health involves not just understanding our body's inherent processes, but also actively nurturing and fortifying it. Central to this nurturing is our diet, the very sustenance that fuels our every cell. But what constitutes a healing diet? Drawing from the foundations of healing nutrition, we delve into the basic principles that transform mere meals into medicinal marvels.

Whole and Unprocessed Foods

At the core of a healing diet lies the emphasis on whole, unprocessed foods. These are foods in their natural or near-natural state, devoid of artificial additives, preservatives, or other synthetic interventions. Examples include fresh fruits and vegetables, whole grains, nuts, seeds, and legumes. Consuming foods in their whole form ensures that we receive a symphony of nutrients, including essential vitamins, minerals, fibres, and antioxidants, which work in harmony to promote health.

Diversity is Key

Just as an orchestra requires a range of instruments to create a harmonious melody, our body thrives on a diverse array of nutrients. Incorporating a wide variety of foods ensures we get a balanced spectrum of micronutrients and macronutrients. This diversity also benefits our gut microbiome, as different microorganisms feed on different dietary components.

Mindful of Macros

While all macronutrients—carbohydrates, proteins, and fats—are vital, the sources and proportions matter. Opt for complex carbohydrates like quinoa, brown rice, and oats over simple sugars. Choose lean proteins like legumes, fish, and poultry, and integrate healthy fats from sources like avocados, nuts, and olive oil.

Hydration for Health

Water is the elixir of life. A healing diet prioritises adequate hydration, understanding that water is crucial for cellular processes, detoxification, digestion, and overall vitality. Infused or herbal waters, herbal teas, and natural broths can also be excellent sources of hydration.

Limiting Inflammatory Foods

Inflammation, when chronic, is the root of many diseases. A healing diet minimises the intake of foods known to cause inflammation. This includes excessive sugary foods, overly processed foods, certain dairy products, and excessive red meats. Instead, it emphasises anti-inflammatory foods like turmeric, berries, green tea, and fatty fish.

Embracing Natural Antioxidants

Antioxidants combat oxidative stress, a major culprit behind ageing and many chronic diseases. Naturally antioxidant-rich foods like blueberries, dark chocolate, spinach, and artichokes should be integral components of a healing diet.

Honouring Personal Needs

A healing diet is not a one-size-fits-all approach. Personalised nutrition, recognizing individual sensitivities, allergies, and metabolic variations, is paramount. It's essential to listen to one's body, consult with health professionals, and tailor dietary choices accordingly.

Conclusion

Embarking on a healing diet is an invitation to reconnect with nature's bounty, to make choices that resonate with our body's innate wisdom. The principles of a healing diet are both simple and profound. They beckon us to return to the basics, prioritise quality over quantity, and nourish ourselves holistically. When we eat with intention, every meal becomes a step toward restoration, rejuvenation, and revitalization.

Essential Nutrients for Optimal Health

The human body, in all its intricacy, operates like a finely tuned machine. But like any machine, it requires specific fuels to run smoothly. These "fuels," or essential nutrients, are compounds our body needs for proper function, growth, and maintenance. Recognizing and incorporating these nutrients is paramount in the journey towards holistic well-being. Here, we delve into these essential nutrients that lay the cornerstone for optimal health.

Macronutrients: The Primary Energy Sources

Carbohydrates: The body's primary energy source, carbohydrates are vital for fueling all our bodily functions. Whole grains, fruits, vegetables, and legumes are excellent sources of beneficial complex carbohydrates.

Proteins: These are vital for tissue repair, hormone production, immune function, and more. Amino acids, the building blocks of proteins, come from dietary sources like lean meats, fish, dairy, eggs, legumes, and certain grains and seeds.

Fats: Crucial for cellular structure, energy, and the absorption of fat-soluble vitamins. Avocados, nuts, seeds, olives, and fatty fish are sources of healthy fats.

Micronutrients: Small but Mighty

Vitamins: These organic compounds are vital for myriad physiological processes: Fat-soluble vitamins (A, D, E, K): Essential for vision, bone health, blood clotting, and antioxidation. Found in foods like dairy, fish, leafy greens, and nuts.

Water-soluble vitamins (C, B complex): Crucial for energy production, immune function, and antioxidation. Found in citrus fruits, whole grains, legumes, and green vegetables.

Minerals: Inorganic nutrients playing a role in bone health, fluid balance, nerve signalling, and more:

Macro-minerals (calcium, potassium, magnesium): Found in dairy products, bananas, nuts, seeds, and leafy greens.

Trace minerals (iron, zinc, iodine, selenium): Found in red meats, seafood, nuts, and whole grains.

Water: The Essence of Life

Comprising about 60% of the human body, water is crucial for nearly every bodily function, including temperature regulation, digestion, and cellular function.

Fibre: For Digestion and Beyond

Dietary fiber, predominantly found in whole grains, fruits, vegetables, and legumes, is essential for optimal digestive health. It also plays roles in weight management, blood sugar stabilisation, and cholesterol reduction.

Omega-3 and Omega-6 Fatty Acids

These essential fatty acids play vital roles in brain health, inflammation regulation, and cell membrane structure. Omega-3s are primarily found in fatty fish, flaxseeds, and walnuts, while Omega-6s are present in vegetable oils, poultry, and eggs.

Phytochemicals: Nature's Medicinal Arsenal

Beyond traditional nutrients, plants offer a vast array of compounds with antioxidant, anti-inflammatory, and disease-fighting properties. Flavonoids, carotenoids, and glucosinolates are just a few examples of phytochemicals found in fruits, vegetables, grains, and teas.

Conclusion

Understanding and integrating these essential nutrients into our daily diets sets the foundation for a life of vitality, resilience, and holistic well-being. Through this knowledge, we don't just feed our bodies; we truly nourish our essence.

The Gut Microbiome: Our Internal Ecosystem

The human body is often likened to a temple, a sacred space requiring reverence and care. But within this temple lies another realm, often overlooked but equally vital: the gut microbiome. This internal ecosystem has profound implications for our health, well-being, and even our emotions. Understanding this complex community of microorganisms offers invaluable insights into the very foundations of healing nutrition.

What is the Gut Microbiome?

Deep within our digestive tract, primarily in the large intestine, resides a bustling community of bacteria, fungi, viruses, and other microorganisms. This collective is the gut microbiome. In sheer numbers, these microbes are staggering, with microbial cells in our body roughly equating to, if not exceeding, our human cells.

The Formative Years

The foundation of our gut microbiome is laid right at birth. Babies born vaginally inherit a set of microbes from their mothers, different from those born via C-section. This microbial profile evolves over time, influenced by factors like breastfeeding, diet, antibiotics, and environmental exposures.

Functions of the Gut Microbiome

Digestion: Certain fibres and compounds, indigestible by human enzymes, are broken down by gut bacteria into short-chain fatty acids. These play pivotal roles in colon health and energy provision.

Immune Modulation: The gut microbiome interacts with our immune cells, training them and modulating their responses.

Vitamin Synthesis: Some gut bacteria are involved in producing vitamins like vitamin K and certain B vitamins.

Neurotransmitter Production: Surprisingly, our gut microbes can produce neurotransmitters, like serotonin, which play roles in mood regulation.

Diet and the Microbiome

What we consume has a direct impact on our microbial community. Diets rich in diverse plant-based foods foster a varied microbiome. In contrast, diets high in processed foods and sugars can reduce microbial diversity. Prebiotics, found in foods like garlic, onions, and asparagus, feed beneficial bacteria. Probiotics, from fermented foods like yoghourt and kimchi, introduce beneficial bacteria.

The Gut-Brain Axis

Emerging research is shining light on the profound connection between the gut and the brain. This gut-brain axis suggests that our gut microbes can influence our emotions, stress responses, and even behaviours.

Implications of an Imbalanced Microbiome

A disrupted gut microbiome, termed dysbiosis, is associated with numerous health issues. These range from gastrointestinal disorders like IBS to metabolic conditions, autoimmune diseases, and even certain mental health conditions.

Nurturing Our Microbial Allies

A holistic approach to health recognizes the importance of nurturing our gut microbes. This involves consuming a balanced, fibre-rich diet, avoiding unnecessary antibiotics, managing stress, and considering probiotic and prebiotic supplementation when appropriate.

Conclusion

Our internal ecosystem, the gut microbiome, is a testament to the interconnectedness of life. It challenges the very notion of individuality, suggesting that our health and well-being are intricately tied to the health of trillions of microorganisms residing within us. By honouring and nurturing this relationship, we tap into a profound source of healing, resilience, and vitality. Our gut microbiome isn't just a part of us; in many ways, it defines us.

Chapter 3: Energising Breakfast Bowls

Quinoa Berry Bliss Bowl

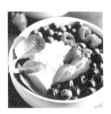

Ingredients

1 cup cooked quinoa

½ cup mixed berries (strawberries, blueberries, raspberries)

2 tbsp chia seeds

1 tbsp honey or maple syrup

¼ cup unsweetened almond milk

A sprinkle of chopped nuts (almonds, walnuts)

Instructions:

Prepare quinoa according to the package instructions. Let it cool to room temperature once cooked.

In a bowl, gently mix the cooked quinoa with almond milk.

Top the quinoa with an assortment of mixed berries.

Evenly sprinkle chia seeds over the berries.

Garnish with a handful of chopped nuts.

Drizzle honey or maple syrup over the entire assembly for added sweetness.

Nutritional Value:

Carbs: 50g

Protein: 12g

Fat: 8g

Fibre: 10g

Tropical Mango & Coconut Bowl

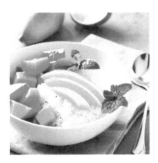

Ingredients:

1 cup diced fresh mango

2 tbsp shredded unsweetened coconut

1 tbsp pumpkin seeds

1 tbsp sunflower seeds

1 cup Greek yoghourt

Instructions:

Lay a base of Greek yoghourt in a deep bowl.

Neatly arrange the diced mango chunks over the yoghourt.

Sprinkle the shredded coconut uniformly over the mango.

Top with pumpkin and sunflower seeds, distributed evenly.

Mix gently before consuming or savour the layers as they are.

Nutritional Value:

Carbs: 45g

Protein: 18g

Fat: 10g

Fibre: 5g

Chia Seed Power Bowl

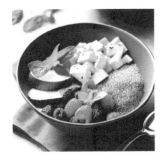

Ingredients:

3 tbsp chia seeds

1 cup unsweetened almond milk

1 sliced banana

2 tbsp almond butter

1 tbsp cocoa nibs

Instructions:

In a medium-sized bowl, combine chia seeds and almond milk. Stir well.

Allow the mixture to sit for at least 20 minutes or until it achieves a gel-like consistency.

Once set, adorn with banana slices, distributing them evenly.

Spoon almond butter on top and sprinkle with cocoa nibs.

Stir gently for a combined texture or eat as layered.

Nutritional Value:

Carbs: 40g

Protein: 10g

Fat: 20g

Fibre: 15g

Savory Veggie & Hummus Bowl

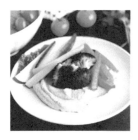

Ingredients:

1 cup roasted vegetables (bell peppers, zucchini, carrots)

2 boiled eggs, halved (chia seed - soaked)

3 tbsp hummus

1 tbsp sesame seeds

Instructions:

Begin by roasting your choice of vegetables in the oven until they're tender.

In a bowl, place your roasted veggies.

Place the halved boiled eggs amongst the veggies.

Add dollops of hummus to the bowl.

Finish by sprinkling sesame seeds over the entire bowl.

Nutritional Value:

Carbs: 20g

Protein: 15g

Fat: 18g

Fibre: 8g

Nutty Avocado Bowl

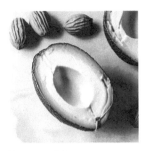

Ingredients:

1 ripe avocado, sliced

1 tbsp flax seeds

1 tbsp hemp seeds

2 tbsp roasted mixed nuts (cashews, almonds, hazelnuts)

A drizzle of extra virgin olive oil

Instructions:

Carefully slice a ripe avocado and place the slices in your bowl.

Sprinkle with flax seeds and hemp seeds for added nutrition.

Add your choice of roasted mixed nuts.

Drizzle a bit of extra virgin olive oil to bring it all together.

Nutritional Value:

Carbs: 12g

Protein: 8g

Fat: 30g

Fibre: 10g

Mediterranean Breakfast Bowl

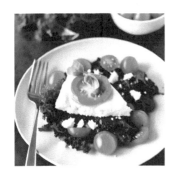

Ingredients:

1 cup sautéed kale

½ cup cherry tomatoes, halved

¼ cup feta cheese, crumbled

¼ cup olives

2 tbsp tzatziki sauce

Instructions:

Sauté kale in a pan with a touch of olive oil until wilted.

Transfer the kale to a bowl and spread it evenly.

Decoratively place halved cherry tomatoes and olives on top.

Sprinkle crumbled feta cheese for a salty kick.

Finish with a generous dollop of tzatziki sauce.

Nutritional Value:

Carbs: 15g

Protein: 10g

Fat: 15g

Fibre: 5g

Tempeh & Greens Breakfast Bowl

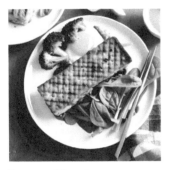

Ingredients:

1 cup sautéed spinach and kale

100g tempeh, grilled

2 tbsp tahini sauce

1 tbsp sunflower seeds

Instructions:

In a skillet, sauté spinach and kale until just wilted. Place them in your bowl.

Grill tempeh slices until they have a nice char and add them to the bowl.

Drizzle over with a rich tahini sauce.

Finish with a sprinkle of sunflower seeds for added crunch.

Nutritional Value:

Carbs: 20g

Protein: 21g

Fat: 15g

Fibre: 6g

Seeded Greek Yogurt Bowl

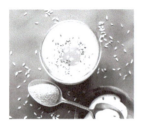

Ingredients:

1 cup ~~Greek~~ coconut yoghourt

1 tbsp flax seeds

1 tbsp chia seeds

1 tbsp pumpkin seeds

1 tbsp honey or maple syrup

Instructions:

Lay a base of creamy Greek yoghourt in your bowl.

Evenly sprinkle flax seeds, chia seeds, and pumpkin seeds on top.

Finish with a drizzle of honey or maple syrup for a touch of sweetness.

Nutritional Value:

Carbs: 30g

Protein: 20g

Fat: 10g

Fibre: 10g

Hearty Chickpea Salad Bowl

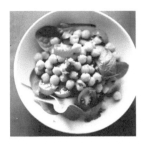

Ingredients:

1 cup chickpeas, boiled and seasoned

1 cucumber, diced

1 carrot, shredded

½ red bell pepper, diced

2 tbsp lemon-tahini dressing

Instructions:

Begin by boiling chickpeas until tender, then season them with your choice of herbs.

In your bowl, mix diced cucumber, shredded carrot, and diced bell pepper.

Add the seasoned chickpeas to the vegetable mix.

Dress with a zesty lemon-tahini sauce.

Nutritional Value:

Carbs: 45g

Protein: 15g

Fat: 10g

Fibre: 12g

Nuts & Berries Greek Yogurt Bowl

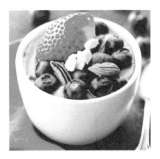

Ingredients:

1 cup Greek yoghourt

½ cup mixed berries

2 tbsp mixed nuts, chopped

1 tbsp honey or maple syrup

Instructions:

Pour Greek yoghourt into your bowl, smoothing it out as a base.

Neatly place a colourful assortment of mixed berries on top.

Sprinkle with a hearty helping of chopped mixed nuts.

Drizzle honey or maple syrup over the top for sweetness.

Nutritional Value:

Carbs: 40g

Protein: 18g

Fat: 10g

Fibre: 5g

Chapter 4: Nourishing Porridges & Overnight Oats

Golden Turmeric Porridge

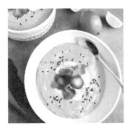

Ingredients:

1 cup ~~rolled oats~~ Buckwheat

2 cups almond milk

1 tsp turmeric powder

A pinch of black pepper

1 tbsp honey or maple syrup

Fresh berries for garnish

Instructions:

Combine rolled oats and almond milk in a saucepan. Cook over medium heat.

As the mixture starts to simmer, add turmeric powder and a pinch of black pepper.

Continue to cook, stirring occasionally, until the oats soften and the mixture thickens.

Remove from heat, sweeten with honey or maple syrup.

Serve in a bowl, garnishing with fresh berries.

Nutritional Value:

Carbs: 55g

Protein: 10g

Fat: 7g

Fibre: 8g

Creamy Coconut & Chia Porridge

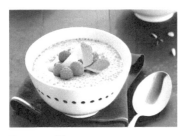

Ingredients:

1 cup ~~rolled oats~~ milk

2 cups coconut milk

2 tbsp chia seeds

1 tbsp shredded coconut

Sliced banana and nuts for topping

Instructions:

Combine rolled oats and coconut milk in a saucepan over medium heat.

Stir in chia seeds as the mixture heats up.

Continue cooking until the oats are tender and the mixture reaches your desired consistency.

Top with sliced banana, nuts, and shredded coconut before serving.

Nutritional Value:

Carbs: 60g

Protein: 12g

Fat: 20g

Fibre: 10g

Cinnamon Apple Porridge

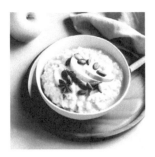

Ingredients:

1 cup ~~rolled oats~~ Quinoa/or millet

2 cups milk of choice

1 apple, diced

1 tsp cinnamon

1 tbsp almond butter

Chopped nuts for garnish

Instructions:

Cook rolled oats with milk in a saucepan over medium heat.

Add diced apple and cinnamon as oats start to soften.

Stir occasionally until oats are cooked through and apples are tender.

Serve warm, drizzling with almond butter and garnishing with chopped nuts.

Nutritional Value:

Carbs: 58g

Protein: 11g

Fat: 9g

Fibre: 9g

Classic Berry ~~Overnight Oats~~ Buckwheat

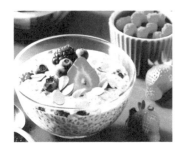

Ingredients:

1 cup ~~rolled oats~~ buckwheat - cooked

1 cup Greek yoghourt

½ cup mixed berries (like blueberries, strawberries, raspberries)

1 tbsp chia seeds

1 cup almond milk

1 tbsp honey or maple syrup

Instructions:

In a jar or bowl, combine ~~rolled oats~~, Greek yoghourt, almond milk, and chia seeds.

Stir well to ensure everything is well-mixed.

Add in your mixed berries, gently folding them in.

Sweeten with honey or maple syrup, then cover the container.

Refrigerate overnight. In the morning, give it a good stir and enjoy!

Nutritional Value:

Carbs: 55g

Protein: 20g

Fat: 7g

Fibre: 10g

Tropical Mango & Coconut ~~Overnight Oats~~ Quinoa

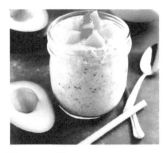

Ingredients:

1 cup ~~rolled oats~~ Quinoa

1 cup coconut milk

½ cup diced mango

1 tbsp shredded coconut

1 tbsp chia seeds

Instructions:

Mix rolled oats, coconut milk, and chia seeds in a bowl or jar.

Add in the diced mango and shredded coconut.

Ensure everything is well combined, then cover the container.

Let it sit in the refrigerator overnight.

Stir and savour in the morning!

Nutritional Value:

Carbs: 52g

Protein: 8g

Fat: 20g

Fibre: 9g

Peanut Butter & Banana Overnight Oats

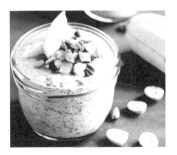

Ingredients:

1 cup ~~rolled oats~~ millet

1 cup almond milk

1 banana, sliced

2 tbsp peanut butter

1 tbsp chia seeds

A drizzle of honey or maple syrup

Instructions:

In a container, combine rolled oats, almond milk, and chia seeds.

Add sliced bananas and dollops of peanut butter.

Mix well to make sure the ingredients are evenly distributed.

Use honey or maple syrup to drizzle for sweetness.

Cover and let it soak overnight in the refrigerator.

Mix and munch in the morning!

Nutritional Value:

Carbs: 60g

Protein: 15g

Fat: 18g

Fibre: 10g

Chocolate Almond Overnight ~~Oats~~ Buckwheat

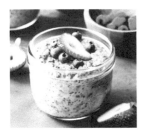

Ingredients:

1 cup ~~rolled oats~~ Buckwheat

1 cup almond milk

2 tbsp cocoa powder

1 tbsp chia seeds

2 tbsp almond slices

1 tbsp honey or maple syrup

Instructions:

In your chosen container, mix rolled oats, almond milk, cocoa powder, and chia seeds.

Ensure cocoa is well dissolved and mixed.

Sweeten with honey or maple syrup and top with almond slices.

Cover and allow the mixture to soak overnight in the refrigerator.

Stir and savour your chocolatey delight in the morning.

Nutritional Value:

Carbs: 58g

Protein: 12g

Fat: 12g

Fibre: 9g

Mixed Berry and Chia Seed Porridge

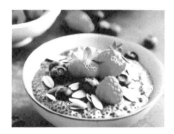

Ingredients:

1/2 cup rolled oats

1 cup almond milk

1/4 cup mixed berries (blueberries, raspberries, strawberries)

2 tsp chia seeds

1 tbsp honey or maple syrup

A pinch of salt

Fresh mint leaves for garnish

Instructions:

In a saucepan, combine the rolled oats and almond milk. Cook over medium heat, stirring occasionally.

As the mixture begins to simmer, add the chia seeds and a pinch of salt.

Continue cooking until the oats are soft and the porridge is creamy, around 5 minutes.

Remove from heat and stir in the honey or maple syrup.

Serve in a bowl topped with mixed berries and garnished with fresh mint leaves.

Nutritional Value:

Calories: 280
Protein: 6g
Fat: 7g
Carbohydrates: 49g
Fibre: 9g

Golden Turmeric Overnight Oats

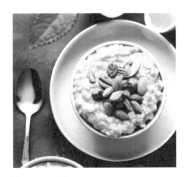

Ingredients:

1/2 cup rolled oats

1 cup coconut milk

1 tsp turmeric powder

1/2 tsp ground cinnamon

1 tbsp chia seeds

1 tbsp honey or maple syrup

A pinch of black pepper

Instructions:

In a mason jar or bowl, mix together the rolled oats, coconut milk, turmeric powder, ground cinnamon, chia seeds, and a pinch of black pepper.

Add the honey or maple syrup whilst stiring for sweetness.

Seal the jar or cover the bowl and refrigerate overnight.

In the morning, give the oats a good stir and add more milk if necessary to reach your desired consistency.

Before serving, top with your favourite fruits or nuts.

Nutritional Value:
Calories: 310
Protein: 7g
Fat: 14g
Carbohydrates: 40g
Fibre: 8g

Creamy Coconut and Date Porridge

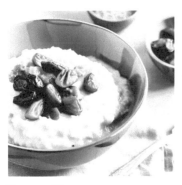

Ingredients:

1/2 cup rolled oats

1 cup coconut milk

3-4 pitted dates, chopped

1 tbsp shredded coconut

1 tbsp flax seeds

1 tsp vanilla extract

A pinch of salt

Instructions:

Combine the rolled oats, coconut milk, and a pinch of salt in a saucepan.

Cook over medium heat, stirring occasionally.

As the mixture starts to simmer, add the chopped dates and flax seeds.

Continue cooking until the oats are soft and have absorbed most of the coconut milk, about 5-7 minutes.

Stir in the vanilla extract and remove from heat.

Serve in a bowl, topped with shredded coconut.

Nutritional Value:
Calories: 320
Protein: 7g
Fat: 15g
Carbohydrates: 42g
Fibre: 8g

Chapter 5: Revitalising Smoothies & Juices

Green Powerhouse Smoothie

Ingredients:

1 cup spinach

1/2 avocado

1 banana

1 tbsp chia seeds

1 cup almond milk

1 tbsp honey

Instructions:

Blend spinach, avocado, banana, chia seeds, and almond milk until smooth.

Sweeten with honey and blend once more.

Pour into a glass and enjoy the rejuvenating blend.

Nutritional Value:

Carbs: 45g

Protein: 8g

Fat: 15g

Fibre: 10g

Berry Bliss Smoothie

Ingredients:

1 cup mixed berries (strawberries, blueberries, raspberries)

1/2 cup Greek yoghourt

1 cup coconut water

1 tbsp flaxseeds

Instructions:

Blend mixed berries, Greek yoghourt, coconut water, and flaxseeds until smooth.

Pour into a glass and savour the fruity goodness.

Nutritional Value:

Carbs: 40g

Protein: 12g

Fat: 5g

Fibre: 8g

Tropical Turmeric Smoothie

Ingredients:

1 cup diced mango

1/2 cup pineapple chunks

1 tsp turmeric powder

1 cup coconut milk

1 tbsp honey

Instructions:

Blend mango, pineapple, turmeric powder, coconut milk until smooth.

Sweeten with honey and blend again.

Pour into a glass and enjoy the tropical vitality.

Nutritional Value:

Carbs: 50g

Protein: 3g

Fat: 10g

Fibre: 5g

Peanut Butter & Banana Smoothie

Ingredients:

1 banana

2 tbsp peanut butter

1 cup almond milk

1 tbsp chia seeds

A drizzle of honey or maple syrup

Instructions:

Blend banana, peanut butter, almond milk, and chia seeds until smooth.

Sweeten with honey or maple syrup and blend again.

Pour into a glass and relish the nutty delight.

Nutritional Value:

Carbs: 40g

Protein: 10g

Fat: 10g

Fibre: 6g

Chocolate Almond Smoothie

Ingredients:

1 banana

1 cup almond milk

2 tbsp cocoa powder

2 tbsp almond butter

1 tbsp honey or maple syrup

Instructions:

Blend banana, almond milk, cocoa powder, almond butter until smooth.

Sweeten with honey or maple syrup and blend once more.

Pour into a glass and enjoy.

Nutritional Value:

Carbs: 45g

Protein: 10g

Fat: 14g

Fibre: 8g

Refreshing Green Juice

Ingredients:

2 cups kale

1 cucumber

2 celery stalks

1 green apple

1/2 lemon

Instructions:

Juice kale, cucumber, celery stalks, green apple.

Squeeze in the lemon juice.

Stir well and serve chilled.

Nutritional Value:

Carbs: 35g

Protein: 4g

Fat: 1g

Fibre: 6g

Sunrise Citrus Juice

Ingredients:

2 oranges, peeled

1 grapefruit, peeled

1 carrot

A slice of ginger

Instructions:

Juice oranges, grapefruit, carrot.

Add a slice of ginger and juice.

Stir to combine and enjoy the citrus burst.

Nutritional Value:

Carbs: 45g

Protein: 3g

Fat: 0.5g

Fibre: 5g

Beetroot Boost Juice

Ingredients:
1 medium beetroot
2 carrots
1 apple
1/2 lemon
Instructions:
Juice beetroot, carrots, and apples.
Squeeze in lemon juice.
Stir well and relish the detoxifying essence.
Nutritional Value: Carbs: 40g
Protein: 2g   Fat: 0.3g
Fibre: 6g

Zesty Ginger Tonic

Ingredients:

1 apple

1 slice ginger

1/2 cucumber

1/2 lemon

Instructions:

Juice apple, ginger, cucumber.

Squeeze in lemon juice.

Stir and serve the invigorating mix.

Nutritional Value:

Carbs: 30g

Protein: 1g

Fat: 0.2g

Fibre: 4g

Chapter 6: Wholesome Salads

Quinoa & Roasted Veggie Salad

Ingredients:

1 cup cooked quinoa

1 cup roasted vegetables (bell peppers, zucchini, broccoli)

1/4 cup feta cheese, crumbled

2 tbsp olive oil

1 tbsp lemon juice

Salt and pepper to taste

Fresh parsley for garnish

Instructions:

In a large mixing bowl, combine cooked quinoa and roasted vegetables.

Over the mixture, drizzle olive oil and lemon juice.

Gently toss until well combined. Season with salt and pepper.

Sprinkle crumbled feta cheese and garnish with fresh parsley before serving.

Nutritional Value:

Carbs: 45g

Protein: 12g

Fat: 15g

Fibre: 8g

Kale & Avocado Bliss Salad

Ingredients:

2 cups kale, chopped

1 avocado, sliced

1/4 cup cherry tomatoes, halved

2 tbsp pumpkin seeds

2 tbsp olive oil

1 tbsp balsamic vinegar

Salt and pepper to taste

Instructions:

In a salad bowl, combine chopped kale, avocado slices, and cherry tomatoes.

Whisk together olive oil and balsamic vinegar in a separate small bowl.

Over the salad, drizzle the dressing and toss to coat.

Top with pumpkin seeds and spice with salt and pepper.

Nutritional Value:

Carbs: 30g

Protein: 8g

Fat: 20g

Fibre: 10g

Chickpea & Spinach Power Salad

Ingredients:

1 cup chickpeas, boiled and drained

2 cups fresh spinach leaves

1/4 cup red onion, finely sliced

1/4 cup feta cheese, crumbled

2 tbsp olive oil

1 tbsp lemon juice

Salt and pepper to taste

Instructions:

Combine chickpeas, fresh spinach leaves, and red onion in a salad bowl.

Drizzle with olive oil and lemon juice.

Toss the salad gently to mix ingredients.

Sprinkle crumbled feta cheese on top and season with salt and pepper.

Nutritional Value:

Carbs: 40g

Protein: 14g

Fat: 15g

Fibre: 12g

Roasted Beet & Goat Cheese Salad

Ingredients:

2 medium beetroots, roasted and sliced

1/4 cup goat cheese, crumbled

2 cups arugula

1/4 cup walnuts, roasted

2 tbsp olive oil

1 tbsp apple cider vinegar

Salt and pepper to taste

Instructions:

Lay a bed of arugula in a serving bowl.

Arrange the roasted beet slices over the arugula.

Crumble goat cheese and scatter roasted walnuts on top.

In a separate bowl, whisk together olive oil and apple cider vinegar. Drizzle over the salad.

Season with salt and pepper.

Nutritional Value:

Carbs: 25g

Protein: 8g

Fat: 18g   Fibre: 7g

Mediterranean Tuna Salad

Ingredients:

1 can tuna, drained (1 can beans, black - rinsed)

1/4 cup black olives, sliced

1/4 cup cherry tomatoes, halved

1/4 cup cucumber, diced

2 tbsp olive oil

1 tbsp lemon juice

Salt and pepper to taste

Fresh parsley for garnish

Instructions:

In a bowl, flake the drained tuna.

Add olives, cherry tomatoes, and cucumber.

Drizzle with olive oil and lemon juice, then gently mix.

Add salt and pepper for seasoning, and garnish with fresh parsley.

Nutritional Value:

Carbs: 15g

Protein: 20g

Fat: 15g

Fibre: 4g

Broccoli & Toasted Almond Salad

Ingredients:

2 cups broccoli florets, lightly steamed

1/4 cup toasted almonds

1/4 cup dried cranberries

2 tbsp feta cheese, crumbled

2 tbsp olive oil

1 tbsp apple cider vinegar

Salt and pepper to taste

Instructions:

In a salad bowl, combine steamed broccoli florets, toasted almonds, and dried cranberries.

Drizzle with olive oil and apple cider vinegar.

Toss the ingredients together gently.

Top with crumbled feta cheese, and spice with salt and pepper.

Nutritional Value:

Carbs: 28g

Protein: 8g

Fat: 14g

Fibre: 7g

Thai Inspired Mango Salad

Ingredients:

1 ripe mango, sliced thinly

1/4 cup red bell pepper, julienned

1/4 cup carrots, julienned

1/4 cup red onion, thinly sliced

2 tbsp fresh cilantro, chopped

2 tbsp lime juice

1 tbsp olive oil

A pinch of chilli flakes

Salt to taste

Instructions:

Combine mango slices, red bell pepper, carrots, and red onion in a bowl.

Drizzle with lime juice and olive oil.

Toss gently to coat.

Sprinkle with chopped cilantro, chilli flakes, and season with salt.

Nutritional Value:
Carbs: 40g
Protein: 2g
Fat: 7g
Fibre: 5g

Cabbage & Sesame Seed Crunch Salad

Ingredients:

2 cups shredded purple cabbage

1/4 cup sesame seeds, toasted

1/4 cup green onions, sliced

2 tbsp sesame oil

1 tbsp rice vinegar

1 tbsp honey

Salt to taste

Instructions:

In a bowl, combine shredded cabbage, toasted sesame seeds, and green onions.

Whisk together sesame oil, rice vinegar, and honey in a separate small bowl.

Over the cabbage mixture, pour the dressing.

Toss to combine, and season with salt.

Nutritional Value:

Carbs: 30g

Protein: 5g

Fat: 9g

Fibre: 6g

Sun-Dried Tomato & Spinach Pasta Salad

Ingredients:

2 cups cooked whole wheat pasta

1/2 cup sun-dried tomatoes, chopped

1 cup fresh spinach

1/4 cup parmesan cheese, grated

2 tbsp olive oil

1 tbsp lemon juice

Salt and pepper to taste

Instructions:

Mix cooked pasta with sun-dried tomatoes and fresh spinach in a large bowl.

In a separate bowl, whisk together olive oil and lemon juice.

Pour the dressing over the pasta mixture and toss.

Garnish with grated parmesan cheese and season with salt and pepper.

Nutritional Value:

Carbs: 50g

Protein: 12g

Fat: 10g

Fibre: 8g

Greek Inspired Chickpea Salad

Ingredients:

1 cup chickpeas, boiled and drained

1/4 cup cucumbers, diced

1/4 cup red onions, diced

1/4 cup cherry tomatoes, halved

2 tbsp olive oil

1 tbsp lemon juice

1/4 cup feta cheese, crumbled

Fresh oregano, for garnish

Salt and pepper to taste

Instructions:

Combine chickpeas, cucumbers, red onions, and cherry tomatoes in a bowl.

Use olive oil and lemon juice to drizzle and mix gently.

Top with crumbled feta cheese and fresh oregano.

Season with salt and pepper.

Nutritional Value:

Carbs: 40g
Protein: 14g
Fat: 15g
Fibre: 12g

Chapter 7: Healing Soups and Stews

Nourishing Bone Broth Soup

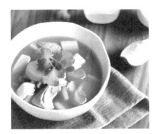

Ingredients:

4 cups bone broth (chicken or beef)

2 carrots, sliced

2 celery stalks, chopped

1 onion, diced

2 cloves garlic, minced

1 bay leaf

Salt and pepper to taste

Instructions:

Begin by washing your carrots and celery. Slice your carrots into rounds and chop the celery stalks into bite-sized pieces. The onion should be diced and minced the garlic.

In a large pot, add your bone broth and heat over medium heat until it starts to simmer.

Incorporate the carrots, celery, onion, and garlic to the simmering broth.

Introduce the bay leaf to the pot. Allow the soup to simmer gently, ensuring the vegetables become tender. This should take about 25-30 minutes.

Before serving, remove the bay leaf. Season the soup with salt and pepper in accordance to your preference.

Dish out the hot soup into bowls and serve immediately.

Creamy Lentil & Spinach Soup

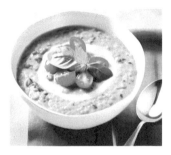

Ingredients:

1 cup lentils, rinsed

4 cups vegetable broth

2 cups spinach leaves

1 onion, diced

1 tbsp olive oil

Salt and pepper to taste

Instructions:

In a pot, heat the olive oil over a medium flame. Incorporate the diced onion and sauté until translucent.

Pour in the vegetable broth. Rinse the lentils and put them in the pot.

Let the soup simmer until lentils are close to being fully cooked.

Gently stir in the spinach leaves, allowing them to wilt into the soup.

Sprinkle some salt and pepper, adjusting to your taste.

Once everything is cooked to perfection, ladle the soup into bowls and enjoy while hot.

Healing Turmeric & Ginger Soup

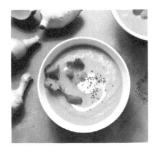

Ingredients:

4 cups chicken broth –

2 carrots, sliced

1 tsp grated ginger

1 tsp turmeric powder

1 chicken breast, diced –

Salt and pepper to taste

Instructions:

Begin by washing and slicing your carrots. Grate the fresh ginger to measure out a teaspoon.

In a pot, heat the chicken broth over medium flame until simmering.

Add the sliced carrots, freshly grated ginger, and turmeric powder to the simmering broth.

Dice the chicken breast and introduce it to the pot. Allow it to cook through.

Season the soup with salt and pepper to your liking.

Pour the soup into bowls, ensuring an even distribution of chicken and carrots. Serve hot.

Immunity-Boosting Mushroom Soup

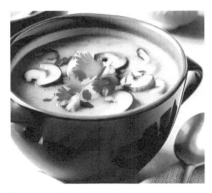

Ingredients:

2 cups mushrooms, sliced

4 cups vegetable broth

1 onion, diced

2 cloves garlic, minced

2 tbsp olive oil

Salt and pepper to taste

Instructions:

In a pot, add olive oil and heat. Add the diced onions and minced garlic, sautéing until they are soft and translucent.

Clean and slice the mushrooms, adding them to the pot. Let them cook until they reduce in size and become tender.

Pour in the vegetable broth, and allow the soup to come to a simmer.

Sprinkle salt and pepper, adjusting according to your taste preference.

Ladle the soup into bowls, making sure to get an even mix of mushrooms and broth in each serving.

Wholesome Vegetable Stew

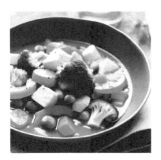

Ingredients:

4 cups mixed vegetables (carrots, potatoes, beans, peas)

4 cups vegetable broth

1 onion, diced

2 tbsp olive oil

2 cloves garlic, minced

Salt and pepper to taste

Instructions:

Start by heating olive oil in a pot. Add the diced onions and minced garlic, letting them become translucent.

Wash and chop the mix of vegetables you have chosen. Add them to the pot, stirring for a few minutes to let them sear slightly.

Pour in the vegetable broth, ensuring it covers the vegetables. Bring the mixture to a boil.

Lower the heat, letting the stew simmer until all the vegetables become tender.

Season with salt and pepper as per your taste.

Dish out generous servings into bowls, ensuring a mix of vegetables in each. Enjoy hot.

Rejuvenating Beet Soup (Borscht)

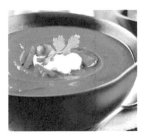

Ingredients:

2 medium beetroots, peeled and diced

1 carrot, diced

1 onion, diced

4 cups beef broth

2 tbsp olive oil

1 tbsp apple cider vinegar

Salt and pepper to taste

Fresh dill for garnish

Instructions:

Begin by peeling and dicing the beetroots and carrots. Meanwhile, dice the onion as well.

In a large pot, warm the olive oil over medium heat. Add the onions and sauté until they are translucent. Introduce the diced beetroots and carrots, cooking them for about 5 minutes.

Pour in the beef broth and increase the heat to bring the mixture to a boil.

Once boiling, reduce the heat and let the soup simmer for about 20 minutes, or until the beetroots and carrots are tender.

Mix in the apple cider vinegar and season with salt and pepper according to your taste.

Ladle the hot soup into bowls, garnishing with freshly chopped dill.

Nutritional Value: Carbs: 20g

Protein: 10g   Fat: 7g

Fibre: 5g

Heart-Warming Pumpkin Soup

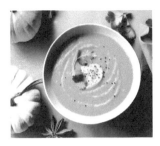

Ingredients:

2 cups pumpkin puree

3 cups vegetable broth

1 onion, diced

1 tsp ground cinnamon

1/2 tsp nutmeg

Salt and pepper to taste

1 tbsp olive oil

Instructions:

In your pot, heat the olive oil over medium heat. Add the diced onion, cooking until it's soft and translucent.

Introduce the pumpkin puree to the pot, followed by the cinnamon and nutmeg. Stir well to combine.

Pour in the vegetable broth and mix thoroughly, ensuring a consistent blend.

Let the soup gently simmer for about 20 minutes, allowing the flavors to meld together.

Add salt and pepper, adjusting to your preference.

Once ready, dish out the soup into bowls, serving it warm.

Nutritional Value: Carbs: 25g

Protein: 4g   Fat: 6g

Fibre: 7g

Revitalising Fish Stew

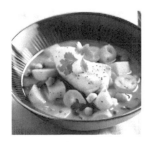

Ingredients:

2 fish fillets (like cod or haddock), diced

4 cups fish broth

1 bell pepper, diced

1 onion, diced

2 cloves garlic, minced

1 tbsp olive oil

Salt and pepper to taste

Instructions:

In your pot, warm the olive oil. Add the diced onion, bell pepper, and minced garlic, sautéing until the onions become translucent.

Pour in the fish broth and bring it to a simmer. Once simmering, add the diced fish fillets.

Allow the fish to cook in the broth until it's fully done and easily flakes.

Season the stew with salt and pepper to your taste.

Ladle the stew into bowls, ensuring each serving has an ample amount of fish and vegetables.

Nutritional Value:

Carbs: 15g

Protein: 20g

Fat: 8g Fibre: 3g

Hearty Chickpea & Tomato Soup

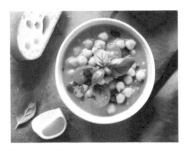

Ingredients:

1 cup chickpeas, soaked and boiled

2 cups tomato puree

4 cups vegetable broth

1 onion, diced

2 cloves garlic, minced

2 tbsp olive oil

1 tsp dried basil

Salt and pepper to taste

Instructions:

Heat olive oil in your pot. Add the diced onion and minced garlic, cooking until the onions are translucent.

Incorporate the tomato puree and the boiled chickpeas to the pot. Stir in the dried basil.

Pour in the vegetable broth, mixing well.

Allow the soup to simmer for approximately 25 minutes, ensuring the chickpeas are tender and flavours are well combined.

Add salt and pepper according to your liking.

Dish out the soup into bowls and enjoy it hot.

Chapter 8: Plant-Powered Main Courses

Stuffed Bell Peppers with Quinoa & Veggies

Ingredients:

4 bell peppers (varied colours)

1 cup cooked quinoa

1 cup black beans, rinsed and drained

1 cup corn kernels

1 onion, diced

2 cloves garlic, minced

2 tbsp olive oil

Salt and pepper to taste

Fresh cilantro for garnish

Instructions:

Begin by preheating your oven to 375°F (190°C). Wash the bell peppers and remove the tops. Clear the seeds and membranes, creating a hollow.

In a skillet, heat olive oil over medium flame. Add diced onion and garlic, sautéing until translucent. Add black beans, corn, and cooked quinoa. Stir well and spice with salt and pepper. Cook until the mixture is heated through.

Stuff each bell pepper with the quinoa mixture, pressing gently to pack the filling.

Place the stuffed peppers in a baking dish. Cover with aluminium foil and bake for about 25-30 minutes, or until the peppers are tender.

Remove from oven and allow to cool slightly. Garnish with fresh cilantro and serve.

Nutritional Value: Carbs: 45g   Protein: 12g

Fat: 8g   Fibre: 10g

Eggplant & Chickpea Curry

Ingredients:

2 medium eggplants, diced

1 can chickpeas, rinsed and drained

1 can coconut milk

2 tbsp curry powder

1 onion, diced

2 cloves garlic, minced

1 tbsp coconut oil

Salt to taste

Fresh coriander for garnish

Instructions:

In a large pan, melt the coconut oil. Add the diced onions and minced garlic, sautéing until they're golden.

Introduce the diced eggplants to the pan and stir until slightly softened. Sprinkle in the curry powder, ensuring the eggplants are well coated.

Pour the coconut milk into the pan and add the chickpeas. Mix well.

Let the mixture come to a gentle simmer. Cook for 20-25 minutes, stirring occasionally until the eggplant is tender and the flavours meld.

Once done, season with salt according to taste. Garnish with fresh coriander leaves and serve warm, ideally with some brown rice or whole grain flatbread.

Nutritional Value:

Carbs: 50g

Protein: 14g

Fat: 20g

Fibre: 12g

Lentil & Vegetable Shepherd's Pie

Ingredients:

1 cup green lentils, rinsed and boiled

3 cups mixed vegetables (carrots, peas, corn)

4 potatoes, boiled and mashed

1 onion, diced

2 cloves garlic, minced

2 tbsp olive oil

Salt and pepper to taste

Instructions:

Start by heating the olive oil in a skillet. Incorporate the diced onion and minced garlic, cooking until they become soft and fragrant.

Incorporate the mixed vegetables and boiled lentils into the skillet. Stir for some minutes until well combined and heated.

In a separate bowl, take your boiled potatoes and mash them until smooth. Spice with a bit of salt and pepper.

In a baking dish, lay out the lentil and vegetable mixture as the base. Smoothly spread the mashed potatoes over the top as the second layer.

Preheat your oven to 375°F (190°C) and bake the pie for 25-30 minutes or until the top is golden and slightly crispy.

Allow it to cool slightly, then slice and serve.

Nutritional Value:

Carbs: 55g

Protein: 18g

Fat: 10g Fibre: 15g

Zucchini Noodle Stir-Fry with Tofu

Ingredients:

4 medium zucchinis, spiralized into noodles

200g firm tofu, cubed

2 bell peppers, thinly sliced

2 tbsp soy sauce

1 tbsp sesame oil

2 cloves garlic, minced

1 tsp grated ginger

1 tbsp olive oil

Instructions:

Begin by pressing the tofu to remove excess water. Cube the tofu into bite-sized pieces.

In a large skillet, heat olive oil over medium heat. Add the tofu cubes, allowing them to brown on all sides. This should take about 5-7 minutes.

Incorporate the sliced bell peppers, minced garlic, and grated ginger into the skillet. Stir well and cook until the peppers are slightly softened. Add the zucchini noodles and drizzle with soy sauce and sesame oil. Toss the ingredients to combine and heat through.

Once everything is well-cooked and flavours are melded, dish out the stir-fry into bowls and serve immediately.

Nutritional Value:

Carbs: 30g

Protein: 14g

Fat: 12g

Fibre: 7g

Cauliflower Steak with Pesto

Ingredients:

2 large cauliflowers, sliced into steaks

2 tbsp olive oil

Salt and pepper to taste

For the Pesto:

1 cup fresh basil leaves

2 cloves garlic

1/4 cup pine nuts

1/3 cup olive oil

Salt to taste

Instructions:

Start by washing the cauliflowers. Slice them into 1-inch thick steaks. Use olive oil to drizzle and season with salt and pepper.

Preheat your grill or a skillet over medium heat. Place the cauliflower steaks and grill/cook until they're tender and have grill marks, approximately 5 minutes on each side.

While the cauliflower is cooking, prepare the pesto. In a food processor, combine basil, garlic, pine nuts, olive oil, and salt. Blend until the paste is smooth

Once the cauliflower steaks are done, plate them. Drizzle or spread the pesto over the steaks. Serve warm.

Nutritional Value:

Carbs: 20g

Protein: 6g

Fat: 18g Fibre: 8g

Chickpea & Spinach Curry

Ingredients:

1 can chickpeas, rinsed and drained

2 cups fresh spinach leaves, washed

1 can coconut milk

2 tbsp curry powder

1 onion, diced

2 cloves garlic, minced

1 tbsp coconut oil

Salt and pepper to taste

Instructions:

In a skillet, melt the coconut oil over medium heat. Add the diced onion and minced garlic, cooking until golden.

Incorporate the chickpeas and curry powder. Stir well to ensure the chickpeas are coated.

Pour in the coconut milk, blending well. Introduce the spinach leaves, allowing them to wilt into the curry.

Let the curry gently simmer for about 15 minutes, making sure the flavors infuse together.

Season with salt and pepper. Dish out the curry into bowls and serve with brown rice or whole grain flatbread.

Nutritional Value:

Carbs: 40g

Protein: 14g

Fat: 18g

Fibre: 10g

Vegan Eggplant Parmesan

Ingredients:

2 large eggplants, sliced

2 cups tomato sauce (homemade or store-bought)

2 cups vegan mozzarella cheese, shredded

1 cup vegan parmesan cheese, grated

1 cup breadcrumbs

2 tbsp olive oil

Salt and pepper to taste

Fresh basil for garnish

Instructions:

Begin by slicing the eggplants into 1/2-inch thick rounds. Season both sides with salt and let them sit for 15 minutes. This helps draw out excess moisture. Wipe them dry.

Dredge the eggplant slices in breadcrumbs, ensuring they are well-coated.

In a skillet, heat the olive oil over medium heat. Cook the breaded eggplant slices until they are golden on both sides. Remove and set aside.

In a baking dish, spread a layer of tomato sauce. Place a layer of the cooked eggplant slices over it. Sprinkle a generous amount of vegan mozzarella and vegan parmesan. Repeat the layers until all the ingredients are finished.

Preheat your oven to 375°F (190°C). Bake the eggplant parmesan until the cheese is melted and bubbly(30 mins approx).

Garnish with fresh basil leaves. Slice and serve warm.

Nutritional Value: Carbs: 45g   Protein: 10g

Fat: 15g   Fibre: 10g

Vegan Lentil Loaf

Ingredients:

2 cups green lentils, cooked

1 onion, diced

2 cloves garlic, minced

1 carrot, grated

2 tbsp olive oil

1 cup breadcrumbs

1/2 cup tomato sauce

2 tbsp soy sauce

1 tbsp flaxseed meal (mixed with 3 tbsp water)

Salt and pepper to taste

Instructions:

In a skillet, heat the olive oil. Add the diced onion, minced garlic, and grated carrot. Cook until the onions are translucent.

In a large bowl, combine cooked lentils, sautéed vegetables, breadcrumbs, half of the tomato sauce, soy sauce, and flaxseed meal mixture. Mix well to make sure all ingredients are combined.

Forming the Loaf: In a loaf pan, press the lentil mixture firmly.

Spread the remaining tomato sauce over the top.

Preheat your oven to 375°F (190°C). Bake the lentil loaf for 40-45 minutes.

Once baked, remove from oven and allow it to cool slightly. Slice and serve.

Nutritional Value:

Carbs: 50g

Protein: 20g

Fat: 10g Fibre: 15g

Vegan Risotto with Asparagus & Mushrooms

Ingredients:

1 cup Arborio rice

4 cups vegetable broth

1 bunch asparagus, chopped

2 cups mushrooms, sliced

1 onion, diced

2 cloves garlic, minced

2 tbsp olive oil

Salt and pepper to taste

Fresh parsley for garnish

Instructions:

In a large pot, heat olive oil. Add diced onion and minced garlic, cooking until translucent. Add the mushrooms and asparagus, sautéing until tender.

Pour in Arborio rice, stirring to coat the rice with the oil and vegetables. Start by adding the vegetable broth, one cup at a time, allowing the rice to absorb the liquid before adding the next.

Continue cooking and stirring, ensuring the rice becomes creamy and fully cooked. Add salt and pepper to season according to your preference.

Dish out the risotto into bowls, garnishing with fresh parsley.

Nutritional Value:

Carbs: 60g

Protein: 8g

Fat: 10g

Fibre: 4g

Vegan Stuffed Acorn Squash

Ingredients:

2 acorn squashes, halved and seeds removed

1 cup wild rice, cooked

1/2 cup cranberries

1/2 cup pecans, chopped

2 tbsp olive oil

Salt and pepper to taste

Maple syrup for drizzling (optional)

Instructions:

Preheat your oven to 400°F (200°C). Drizzle olive oil over the acorn squash halves and season with salt and pepper. On a baking sheet, Place them face down.

Cook the squashes in the preheated oven for about 25-30 minutes or until tender.

In a bowl, combine cooked wild rice, cranberries, and chopped pecans. Spice with salt and pepper, and mix well.

Once the squashes are cooked, flip them over. With the wild rice mixture, fill each squash half.

Return the stuffed squashes to the oven for an additional 10 minutes.

Once done, remove from the oven. Drizzle with maple syrup if desired and serve warm.

Nutritional Value:

Carbs: 65g

Protein: 6g

Fat: 12g

Fibre: 8g

Chapter 9: Comforting One-Pot Dinner Meals

Tuscan White Bean & Kale Stew

Ingredients:

2 cans white beans, rinsed and drained

4 cups kale, chopped

4 cups vegetable broth

1 onion, diced

2 cloves garlic, minced

1 can diced tomatoes

2 tbsp olive oil

Salt and pepper to taste

Red pepper flakes (optional)

Fresh rosemary for garnish

Instructions:

In a large pot, warm olive oil over medium heat. Add the diced onions and minced garlic, sautéing until translucent.
Beans, Tomatoes, and Broth: Stir in the white beans and diced tomatoes. Pour in the vegetable broth and increase heat to bring the mixture to a simmer.
Fold in the chopped kale, ensuring it's submerged in the liquid.
Add salt, pepper, and optional red pepper flakes to taste.
Allow the stew to simmer for about 20-25 minutes, ensuring the kale is tender and flavours melded.
Dish out the stew into bowls, garnishing with fresh rosemary.

Nutritional Value:

Carbs: 45g
Protein: 15g Fat: 7g
Fibre: 11g

One-Pot Vegetable & Chickpea Curry

Ingredients:

1 can chickpeas, rinsed and drained

4 cups mixed vegetables (like bell peppers, carrots, and zucchini), chopped

1 can coconut milk

3 tbsp curry paste

1 onion, diced

2 cloves garlic, minced

2 tbsp coconut oil

Salt to taste

Fresh cilantro for garnish

Instructions:

In a large pot, melt the coconut oil over medium heat. Add the diced onions and minced garlic, sautéing until golden brown.

Add the chopped vegetables and chickpeas, stirring to combine.

Mix in the curry paste, ensuring the veggies and chickpeas are well-coated. Pour in the coconut milk whilst stirring well.

Let the curry gently simmer for 25-30 minutes until the vegetables are tender and the flavours infused.

Adjust the taste with salt.

Dish out the curry into bowls, garnishing with fresh cilantro. Serve with brown rice or quinoa.

Nutritional Value: Carbs: 50g

Protein: 12g Fat: 20g

Fibre: 10g

One-Pot Vegan Chili

Ingredients:

2 cans black beans, rinsed and drained

1 can kidney beans, rinsed and drained

4 cups vegetable broth

1 bell pepper, diced

1 zucchini, diced

1 can diced tomatoes

1 onion, diced

2 cloves garlic, minced

2 tbsp olive oil

2 tbsp chilli powder

Salt and pepper to taste

Fresh parsley for garnish

Instructions:

In a large pot, heat the olive oil. Add the onion and garlic, sautéing until it soft.

Incorporate the bell pepper, zucchini, black beans, and kidney beans.

Pour in the vegetable broth and diced tomatoes. Sprinkle in the chilli powder, salt, and pepper, mixing well.

Let the chilli simmer for about 30-35 minutes, ensuring flavors are well combined and vegetables are tender.

Spoon the chilli into bowls, garnishing with fresh parsley.

Nutritional Value: Carbs: 55g Protein: 18g

Fat: 10g

Fibre: 15g

One-Pot Lentil & Mushroom Stroganoff

Ingredients:

1 cup green lentils, rinsed and boiled

2 cups mushrooms, sliced

1 onion, diced

2 cloves garlic, minced

4 cups vegetable broth

1 cup vegan sour cream

2 tbsp olive oil

Salt and pepper to taste

Fresh parsley for garnish

Instructions:

In a pot, heat the olive oil. Incorporate the onion and garlic, cooking until they are translucent.

Add the sliced mushrooms, allowing them to soften. Introduce the boiled green lentils to the pot.

Pour in the vegetable broth, ensuring the ingredients are well submerged.

Simmer: Allow the mixture to simmer for about 20-25 minutes.

Once the lentils are fully cooked and the flavors melded, stir in the vegan sour cream. Mix until you achieve a creamy consistency.

Season with salt and pepper. Ladle the stroganoff into bowls, garnishing with fresh parsley.

Nutritional Value: Carbs: 50g

Protein: 20g   Fat: 10g

Fibre: 15g

Mediterranean One-Pot Orzo & Veggies

Ingredients:

1 cup orzo pasta

2 cups cherry tomatoes, halved

1 bell pepper, diced

1 zucchini, diced

4 cups vegetable broth

1 onion, diced

2 cloves garlic, minced

1 cup Kalamata olives, pitted and sliced

2 tbsp olive oil

Salt and pepper to taste

Fresh basil for garnish

Instructions:

In a pot, heat olive oil. Add onions and garlic, sautéing until golden brown.

Incorporate the bell pepper, zucchini, and cherry tomatoes, stirring for a few minutes.

Add the orzo to the pot, followed by the vegetable broth. Ensure the orzo is fully submerged.

Let the mixture simmer until the orzo is cooked and has absorbed most of the broth.

Stir in the sliced Kalamata olives. Season with salt and pepper.

Dish out the orzo into bowls, garnishing with fresh basil leaves.

Nutritional Value: Carbs: 60g   Protein: 10g

Fat: 12g   Fibre: 7g

Vegan Spanish Paella

Ingredients:

1 cup Arborio rice

2 cups vegetable broth

1 bell pepper, diced

1 cup green peas

1 cup artichoke hearts, quartered

1 onion, diced

2 cloves garlic, minced

1/4 tsp saffron threads (or turmeric for color)

2 tbsp olive oil

Salt and pepper to taste

Lemon wedges and parsley for garnish

Instructions:

Heat the olive oil in a large skillet or paella pan. Incorporate the diced onion and minced garlic whilst cooking until translucent.

Stir in the Arborio rice, ensuring it's coated with oil. Add the saffron threads or turmeric, mixing well.

Incorporate the bell pepper, green peas, and artichoke hearts. Pour in the vegetable broth, ensuring the rice is submerged.

Allow the mixture to simmer until the rice is tender and has absorbed most of the broth, stirring occasionally.

Once cooked, season with salt and pepper. Serve the paella with lemon wedges and a sprinkle of fresh parsley.

Nutritional Value: Carbs: 65g   Protein: 8g

Fat: 10g   Fibre: 6g

Creamy Vegan One-Pot Pasta

Ingredients:

2 cups ~~whole wheat~~ _Rice_ pasta

4 cups almond milk

1 cup cherry tomatoes, halved

1 cup spinach, chopped

1 onion, diced

2 cloves garlic, minced

2 tbsp nutritional yeast

2 tbsp olive oil

Salt and pepper to taste

Instructions:

In a pot, heat the olive oil. Add the onion and garlic, cooking until soft and fragrant.

Add the pasta to the pot, followed by the almond milk. Make sure the pasta is submerged in the liquid.

Let the pasta cook in the almond milk, stirring occasionally to prevent sticking.

Once the pasta is nearly done, add the cherry tomatoes and spinach, cooking until the spinach wilts.

Stir in the nutritional yeast to give a creamy texture and cheesy flavour.

Season with salt and pepper. Serve the creamy pasta hot, straight from the pot.

Nutritional Value:

Carbs: 70g

Protein: 12g

Fat: 9g

Fibre: 8g

One-Pot Moroccan Chickpea Tagine

Ingredients:

1 can chickpeas, rinsed and drained

4 cups vegetable broth

1 carrot, sliced

1 zucchini, diced

2 tbsp tomato paste

1 onion, diced

2 cloves garlic, minced

2 tbsp olive oil

2 tsp ras el hanout (Moroccan spice blend)

Salt and pepper to taste

Instructions:

In a pot or tagine, heat the olive oil. Add the onion and garlic whilst sautéing until translucent.

Introduce the carrot and zucchini. Stir in the ras el hanout and cook for a couple of minutes.

Add the chickpeas and tomato paste, ensuring everything is well-mixed. Pour in the vegetable broth.

Allow the tagine to simmer for 30-35 minutes, ensuring vegetables are tender and flavours melded.

Season with salt and pepper, then dish out the tagine into bowls, ideally accompanied by couscous.

Nutritional Value: Carbs: 55g Protein: 15g

Fat: 10g Fibre: 12g

One-Pot Vegan Jambalaya

Ingredients:

1 cup brown rice

3 cups vegetable broth

1 bell pepper, diced

1 onion, diced

2 celery stalks, chopped

1 can diced tomatoes

1 cup vegan sausage, sliced

2 tbsp olive oil

2 tsp Cajun seasoning

Salt and pepper to taste

Instructions:

In a pot, heat the olive oil. Add the onion, bell pepper, and celery, cooking until soft.

Stir in the brown rice, ensuring it's coated in the mixture. Add the diced tomatoes and vegan sausage slices.

Pour in the vegetable broth, then sprinkle the Cajun seasoning. Stir well.

Cover the pot and allow the jambalaya to simmer until the rice is fully cooked and has absorbed most of the broth.

Season with salt and pepper. Dish out the jambalaya into bowls and enjoy.

Nutritional Value:

Carbs: 60g

Protein: 10g

Fat: 9g

Fibre: 6g

Vegan Potato & Leek Soup

Ingredients:

4 large potatoes, peeled and diced

2 leeks, cleaned and thinly sliced

4 cups vegetable broth

1 onion, diced

2 cloves garlic, minced

2 tbsp olive oil

Salt and pepper to taste

Instructions:

In a pot, warm the olive oil. Add the onion and garlic, sautéing until they're translucent.

Add the diced potatoes and thinly sliced leeks to the pot, stirring for a few minutes.

Pour in the vegetable broth, ensuring the veggies are submerged.

Let the soup simmer until the potatoes are tender, roughly 25-30 minutes.

For a creamy texture, use a hand blender to blend the soup until smooth, or you can leave it chunky.

Serve

Chapter 10: 28-Day Meal Plan

Combine Lunch/Dinner

Week 1

Day 1:

Pg 25

Breakfast: Quinoa Berry Bliss Bowl

Lunch: Leafy Green Salad with Roasted Chickpeas and Avocado

Dinner: Zucchini Noodle Stir-Fry with Tofu

Dessert: Revitalising Blueberry Almond Smoothie

Day 2:

26

Breakfast: Tropical Mango and ~~Pineapple~~ Coconut Bowl

Lunch: Rainbow Vegetable Salad with Lemon Tahini Dressing

Dinner: Cauliflower Steak with Pesto

Dessert: Refreshing Cucumber Mint Juice

Day 3:

27

Breakfast: ~~Almond Butter & Banana Chia Bowl~~ (Chia Seed Power Bowl)

Lunch: Mediterranean Chickpea Salad with Olives and Feta

Dinner: Chickpea & Spinach Curry

Dessert: Strawberry Banana Bliss Smoothie

Day 4:

28

Breakfast: ~~Hearty Mixed Nuts and Seeds Bowl~~ Savory Vege + Hummus Bowl

Lunch: Tangy Asian Slaw with Crispy Tofu

Dinner: Vegan Eggplant Parmesan

Dessert: Zesty Orange Carrot Juice

Day 5:

29 Breakfast: ~~Spiced Apple and Walnut Delight Bowl~~ (nutty avocado Bowl)

Lunch: Protein-Packed Quinoa and Black Bean Salad

Dinner: Vegan Lentil Loaf

Dessert: Green Goddess Detox Smoothie

30 **Day 6:**

Breakfast: ~~Coconut and Pineapple Sunrise Bowl~~ (mediterranean B.F Bowl)

Lunch: Fresh Fiesta Corn Salad with Lime Dressing

Dinner: Vegan Risotto with Asparagus & Mushrooms

Dessert: Invigorating Beetroot Ginger Juice

31 **Day 7:**

Breakfast: ~~Warm Millet and Berry Morning Bowl~~ (Tempeh and greens B.F Bowl)

Lunch: Hearty Roasted Vegetable Salad with Arugula

Dinner: Vegan Stuffed Acorn Squash

Dessert: Creamy Avocado Lime Smoothie

Week 2

Day 8:

32 Breakfast: ~~Cinnamon Oat & Berry Delight Bowl~~ (Seeded Coconut Yogurt Bowl)

Lunch: Spinach and Feta Couscous Salad

Dinner: Tuscan White Bean & Kale Stew

Dessert: Antioxidant Berry Boost Juice

Day 9:

33 Breakfast: ~~Toasted Coconut & Tropical Fruit Bowl~~ (Hearty Chickpea Salad Bowl)

Lunch: Refreshing Greek Salad with Hummus Dressing

Dinner: One-Pot Vegetable & Chickpea Curry

Dessert: Nutty Chocolate Delight Smoothie

Day 10:

34 Breakfast: ~~Honey Drizzled Peach and Granola Bowl~~ (nuts/Berries Coconut Yogurt Bowl)

Lunch: Protein-Packed Lentil and Farro Salad

Dinner: One-Pot Vegan Chili

Dessert: Energising Apple Celery Juice

Day 11:

35 Breakfast: ~~Lush Fig and Almond Butter Bliss Bowl~~ (Golden Tumeric Porridge)

Lunch: Crispy Kale Caesar Salad with Avocado and Chickpeas

Dinner: One-Pot Lentil & Mushroom Stroganoff

Dessert: Pineapple Mango Tango Smoothie

Day 12:

36 Breakfast: ~~Citrus Burst Breakfast Bowl with Oranges and Grapefruit~~ (Creamy Coconut + Chia Porridge)

Lunch: Warm Beetroot and Quinoa Salad

Dinner: One-Pot Vegan Jambalaya

Dessert: Ruby Red Rejuvenation Juice

Day 13:

37 Breakfast: ~~Toasted Seeds and Honey Crunch Bowl~~ (Cinnamon Apple Porridge)

Lunch: Crunchy Broccoli Slaw with Tangy Dressing

Dinner: Vegan Spanish Paella

Dessert: Berry Bliss Fusion Smoothie

38 **Day 14:**

Breakfast: ~~Banana and Pecan Morning Delight Bowl~~ (Classic Berry, Buckwheat)

Lunch: Spicy Southwest Salad with Corn and Black Beans

Dinner: Creamy Vegan One-Pot Pasta

Dessert: Citrus Sunshine Elixir Juice

Week 3

Day 15:

39 Breakfast: Chocolate Drizzle Raspberry Bowl (Tropical Mango + coconut)

Lunch: Charred Veggie Salad with Zesty Lemon Dressing

Dinner: One-Pot Moroccan Chickpea Tagine

Dessert: Vibrant Berry Beet Smoothie

Day 16:

40 Breakfast: Berry and Walnut Nourish Bowl (Peanut Butter + Banana)

Lunch: Crunchy Thai Salad with Peanut Dressing

Dinner: Healing Tomato and Red Lentil Soup

Dessert: Tropical Pineapple and Coconut Juice

Day 17:

42 Breakfast: Nutty Crunch Bowl with Almonds and Hazelnuts (mixed Berry/chia seed)

Lunch: Mixed Bean Salad with Cilantro-Lime Dressing

Dinner: Asian-Inspired Vegetable Broth with Tofu

Dessert: Green Revitalizer Juice

Day 18:

41 Breakfast: Mango & Chia Seed Energy Bowl (chocolate almond)

Lunch: Mediterranean Tabbouleh Salad with Fresh Herbs

Dinner: Hearty Bean and Vegetable Casserole

Dessert: Refreshing Watermelon and Mint Smoothie

Day 19:

43 Breakfast: Berry Fusion Bowl with Mixed Berries (Golden Turmeric)

Lunch: Waldorf Salad with Creamy Yogurt Dressing

Dinner: Butternut Squash and Lentil Curry

Dessert: Golden Turmeric and Ginger Juice

Day 20:

44 Breakfast: Pineapple & Toasted Coconut Morning Bowl (Creamy Coconut + date)

Lunch: Spinach and Roasted Vegetable Salad with Balsamic Glaze

Dinner: Vegetable and Chickpea Tagine

Dessert: Nutrient-Packed Kale and Spinach Smoothie

Day 21:

45 Breakfast: Honey & Fig Morning Delight Bowl (Green Powerhouse Smoothie)

Lunch: Caesar Salad with Crunchy Croutons and Vegan Caesar Dressing

Dinner: Ratatouille with Fresh Herbs

Dessert: Exotic Mango and Passionfruit Juice

Week 4

Day 22:

Breakfast: Berry & Greek Yogurt Breakfast Bowl (Berry Bliss Smoothie)

Lunch: Thai Green Papaya Salad with Tangy Dressing

Dinner: Vegan Mushroom and Spinach Lasagna

Dessert: Antioxidant-Rich Acai and Blueberry Smoothie

Day 23:

Breakfast: Pear and Granola Energy Boost Bowl (Refreshing Green juice)

Lunch: Roasted Butternut Squash and Arugula Salad with Feta

Dinner: Spicy Vegetable and Bean Chili

Dessert: Revitalising Ruby Red Grapefruit Juice

Day 24:

Breakfast: Mixed Fruit Bowl with Kiwi, Pineapple, and Strawberries (repeat)

Lunch: Grilled Vegetable Salad with Quinoa

Dinner: Vegan Shepherd's Pie with Lentils

Dessert: Berry Infusion Bliss Smoothie

Day 25:

Breakfast: Almond Butter and Blueberry Power Bowl (Repeat)

Lunch: Fresh Mediterranean Salad with Olives and Sundried Tomatoes

Dinner: Vegan Thai Green Curry with Vegetables

Dessert: Cucumber and Lime Hydration Juice

Day 26:

Breakfast: Tropical Fruit Bowl with Dragon Fruit and Mango (Repeat)

Lunch: Fresh Spring Salad with Asparagus and Radishes

Dinner: Vegan Spaghetti with Marinara Sauce and Vegan Meatballs

Dessert: Sweet Pineapple and Basil Smoothie

Day 27:

Breakfast: Chocolate and Raspberry Indulgence Bowl (Repeat)

Lunch: Greek Salad with Cucumbers, Tomatoes, and Vegan Feta

Dinner: Creamy Vegan Potato and Leek Soup

Dessert: Orange, Carrot, and Ginger Zing Juice

Day 28:

Breakfast: Super Seed Bowl with Pumpkin, Sunflower, and Chia Seeds (Repeat)

Lunch: Crunchy Asian Salad with Crispy Noodles and Peanut Dressing

Dinner: Vegetable Stir-Fry with Tofu and Soy Sauce

Dessert: Creamy Banana and Vanilla Smoothie

Crafting a Year-Long Meal Journey: A Blueprint for Wholesome Living

Embracing a year of mindful eating might initially seem daunting, but with the 70 carefully crafted recipes in this book, you're armed with a diverse culinary arsenal. This blueprint will guide you on distributing these recipes across 365 days, ensuring variety, seasonality, and simplicity.

Rotation and Repetition: With 70 recipes, you can comfortably rotate them multiple times throughout the year. This rotation not only eases meal planning but also provides the comfort of familiar favourites. Aim to rotate the recipes roughly five times throughout the year.

Seasonal Adjustments: Certain recipes will resonate more with specific seasons. Fresh salads might be summer staples, while hearty soups and stews warm the heart in winter. Assign recipes to seasons where they fit best, and adjust accordingly. For example, "Hearty Bean and Vegetable Casserole" might be perfect for autumn and winter, while "Leafy Green Salad with Roasted Chickpeas and Avocado" shines in spring and summer.

Monthly Themes: Each month can have a theme based on a specific type of meal or a dominant ingredient. For instance, March can be "Mediterranean March," where Mediterranean-inspired recipes are on the front line. This approach not only adds fun to the meal planning but also ensures that each month has its own distinct flavour.

Weekly Structures: Divide your recipes into categories like breakfast, lunch, dinner, and dessert. Now, structure your week around these. For example, Monday dinners might be one-pot meals, while Wednesdays might focus on plant-powered mains. Fridays can be soup nights, and Sundays dedicated to special breakfast bowls.

Keeping It Fresh: While repetition provides a structure, innovation keeps things exciting. Every 2-3 months, challenge yourself to mix two recipes or incorporate a new ingredient. These minor changes can refresh an old recipe and provide a renewed culinary experience.

Intuitive Adjustments: Listen to your body. There might be days when you crave the comforting warmth of the "Vegan Risotto with Asparagus & Mushrooms" or times when only the "Revitalising Blueberry Almond Smoothie" will do. Allow room for flexibility.

Document and Reflect: Maintain a food journal. Note down which recipes you loved, which ones you tweaked, and how certain meals made you feel. This reflection ensures that by the end of the year, you'll have a deeply personalised version of this meal plan tailored to your tastes and experiences.

Community and Sharing: Make meals a communal experience. Share your dishes with friends or family and gather feedback. This shared experience can offer new insights, alterations, and might even introduce you to new recipes to add to your rotation.

Special Days: For holidays, birthdays, or special occasions, pick out your favorites from the book. These standout recipes will make these days even more memorable.

Remember The Fluidity: This blueprint is a guideline, not a rigid structure. Life is unpredictable, and spontaneity can often lead to the most delightful meals. Embrace changes, and most importantly, enjoy the journey of 'self-healing by design'.

By adopting this blueprint, not only will you navigate through the year with a holistic and varied meal approach, but you'll also deepen your relationship with food, understanding its power to heal, nourish, and bring joy.

1500 Days of Recipes: Mastering the Art of Culinary Variation

A journey of 1500 days starts with a single recipe. Such a statement might seem hyperbolic, but within the culinary world, it encapsulates the essence of creativity, innovation, and versatility. This chapter unveils a unique blueprint that showcases how you can take any one of the 70 foundational recipes in this book and reimagine it in 15 diverse ways. The result? A staggering 1500 days of sumptuous, varied meals.

Why 15 Variations?

Think of each recipe as a beautiful canvas, and the ingredients as your palette. Just as an artist can recreate countless scenes on the same canvas size, so too can you reinterpret a recipe. These 15 variations consider seasonality, available ingredients, cultural inspirations, and dietary preferences.

Here's your blueprint for culinary variety:

Seasonal Twists: A single recipe can shift with the seasons. Fresh berries dominate in summer, root vegetables in winter, tender greens in spring, and hearty squashes in the fall. One recipe, four seasonal avatars.

Cultural Fusion: Take a recipe and reimagine it through a global lens. Add some soy sauce, ginger, and swap in bok choy for a taste of Asia. Or, infuse it with cumin, coriander, and serve over couscous for a Middle Eastern touch.

Dietary Adaptations: Whether you're catering to vegetarians, vegans, or pescatarians, every recipe can be tweaked to align with specific diets. Swap out proteins, introduce new plant-based heroes, or adjust the base.

Texture Play: The same set of ingredients can feel entirely different with texture variations. A creamy soup one day could be a chunky stew the next, or a roasted vegetable salad could turn into a smooth purée.

Herb & Spice Experiments: Introduce a new herb or spice to completely transform the dish. Basil today, tarragon tomorrow. Turmeric in one version, saffron in another.

Sauce Swaps: Change the sauce or dressing, and you instantly have a new dish. A tomato-based dish might get a tangy twist with a tamarind infusion or a creamy depth with a cashew sauce.

Cooking Techniques: Grilled, roasted, steamed, raw – how you prepare your ingredients can introduce new flavours and textures.

Meal Shifts: A dinner recipe could be adapted into a hearty breakfast or a light lunch with some creative tweaks.

Ingredient Exchanges: Swap out a primary ingredient for another star player. If a dish revolves around zucchini, try eggplant the next time.

Presentation Makeovers: Sometimes, a change in presentation can feel like a new meal altogether. A layered dish might be deconstructed the next time.

Portion Adjustments: Turn mains into starters, or starters into mains by playing with portion sizes and accompaniments.

Temperature Changes: A cold salad could be a warm sauté the next day. A hot soup might be a chilled version in summer.

Add-ins and Toppings: Introduce nuts, seeds, dried fruits, or fresh herbs as toppings to change the dish's profile.

Re-imagine Leftovers: Leftovers from one variation could be the start of the next dish.

Community Input: Host tasting sessions and gather feedback. Someone's suggestion might birth the next variation.

With this blueprint in hand, you'll never feel the monotony of repetition. Instead, you'll be embarking on a 1500-day culinary journey, where each day is a new flavour, a new experience, yet rooted in the foundational principles of "Self Heal by Design Diet". Embrace the journey, and let every meal be a testament to creativity and wellness.

Conclusion: Nourishing Your Way to Wellness

As we draw the curtain on the "Self Heal by Design Diet Cookbook," let's pause to appreciate the culinary and healing voyage we've undertaken together. This book has been about more than just recipes; it's been a guide to understanding the profound relationship between our food and our well-being. With every chapter, we've aimed to bridge the space between nutrition, flavour, and the body's intrinsic power to rejuvenate and heal.

Each of the 70 recipes within these pages serves as a testament to the philosophy that our kitchen can be a sanctuary of health, regeneration, and delight. Through meal plans spanning from a month to a transformative 1500-day journey, we've explored the boundless possibilities that arise when we craft meals with intention, knowledge, and passion.

The core essence of the "Self Heal by Design Diet Cookbook" is to instil the understanding that nourishment goes beyond mere sustenance. It's a profound act of self-care, an ode to our body's incredible design, and a celebration of nature's bounty. Every ingredient suggestion, every meal blueprint, and every culinary tip has been curated with the aspiration to guide you closer to a lifestyle that embraces holistic health and well-being.

As you move forward, beyond the confines of this book, carry with you its essence. Let your kitchen be a space where creativity flourishes, where ingredients transform into healing meals, and where each culinary choice becomes a step toward wellness.

Thank you for allowing the "Self Heal by Design Diet Cookbook" to be a part of your healing journey. Remember, true well-being is a harmonious blend of mind, body, and soul. And often, it starts with the choices we make in our kitchens. Here's to a life of health, happiness, and delectable meals!

Bonus: Meal Planning Journal

This journal is designed to complement The Heal By Design Diet Cookbook, offering a space to document, reflect upon, and immerse yourself in the culinary journey towards longevity and vibrant health. Here's a guide on how to make the most of this journal:

The Three-Column Approach:

Each page is structured with three distinct columns to help you organise and record your meals:

Date: Log the day you're having the meal. This not only helps track your culinary journey but also aids in identifying patterns or preferences over time.

Meal: Here, specify which meal of the day the recipe pertains to - Breakfast, Lunch, Dinner, or Snack. This assists in maintaining a balanced intake throughout the day.

Recipe: Write down the name of the recipe you've chosen from the cookbook. This becomes a quick reference point if you wish to revisit or modify the recipe in the future.

Note: Depending on your convenience and the space you require, you can choose to record between 1 to 3 entries per line. This flexible format ensures that the journal adapts to your needs, rather than the other way around.

Recipe Reflections:

Beneath the three columns on each page, there's a dedicated space titled "Recipe Reflections". This is where the journal truly becomes personal:

Feedback: Jot down your thoughts on the recipe you tried. Did it resonate with your palate? Was there a particular flavour that stood out?

Modifications: Did you make any tweaks? Perhaps you added an ingredient or adjusted the cooking method. This space is perfect for noting those customizations for future reference.

Revisit: Would you make the dish again? If so, what might you do differently next time?

Emotional Notes: How did the meal make you feel? Refreshed, energetic, satisfied? Food impacts more than just our physical health, and these emotional notes can help pinpoint meals that uplift your spirit.

Tips for Maximising Your Journal Experience:

Consistency: Try to fill in the journal daily. The more consistent you are, the more valuable and insightful your reflections become.

Honesty: This journal is for you. Be candid with your reflections. The more honest you are about what you liked or didn't, the more tailored and enjoyable your culinary journey will be.

Engage with the Cookbook: Use the journal hand in hand with The Recipes of this book. The two together become a powerful tool, guiding you seamlessly through your optimal health quest.

DATE	MEAL	RECIPE

Recipe Reflections

_____
_____
_____
_____
_____

DATE	MEAL	RECIPE

Recipe Reflections

_____
_____
_____
_____
_____
_____

DATE	MEAL	RECIPE

Recipe Reflections

DATE	MEAL	RECIPE

Recipe Reflections

_____

_____

_____

_____

_____

_____

DATE	MEAL	RECIPE

Recipe Reflections

DATE	MEAL	RECIPE

Recipe Reflections

DATE	MEAL	RECIPE

Recipe Reflections

_____
_____
_____
_____
_____
_____

DATE	MEAL	RECIPE

Recipe Reflections

_____

_____

_____

_____

_____

_____

DATE	MEAL	RECIPE

Recipe Reflections

_____

_____

_____

_____

_____

_____

DATE	MEAL	RECIPE

Recipe Reflections

_____

_____

_____

_____

_____

_____

DATE	MEAL	RECIPE

Recipe Reflections

_____

_____

_____

_____

_____

_____

DATE	MEAL	RECIPE

Recipe Reflections

_____

_____

_____

_____

_____

_____

DATE	MEAL	RECIPE

Recipe Reflections

_____

_____

_____

_____

_____

_____

DATE	MEAL	RECIPE

Recipe Reflections

_____
_____
_____
_____
_____
_____

DATE	MEAL	RECIPE

Recipe Reflections

DATE	MEAL	RECIPE

Recipe Reflections

_____

_____

_____

_____

_____

_____

DATE	MEAL	RECIPE

Recipe Reflections

_____
_____
_____
_____
_____
_____

DATE	MEAL	RECIPE

Recipe Reflections

DATE	MEAL	RECIPE

Recipe Reflections

_____

_____

_____

_____

_____

_____

DATE	MEAL	RECIPE

Recipe Reflections

_____

_____

_____

_____

_____

DATE	MEAL	RECIPE

Recipe Reflections

_____

_____

_____

_____

_____

_____

DATE	MEAL	RECIPE

Recipe Reflections

_____

_____

_____

_____

_____

_____

DATE	MEAL	RECIPE

Recipe Reflections

_____
_____
_____
_____
_____
_____

DATE	MEAL	RECIPE

Recipe Reflections

_____

_____

_____

_____

_____

_____

DATE	MEAL	RECIPE

Recipe Reflections

_____

_____

_____

_____

_____

DATE	MEAL	RECIPE

Recipe Reflections

_____

_____

_____

_____

_____

_____

DATE	MEAL	RECIPE

Recipe Reflections

_____

_____

_____

_____

_____

DATE	MEAL	RECIPE

Recipe Reflections

_____
_____
_____
_____
_____
_____

DATE	MEAL	RECIPE

Recipe Reflections

_____

_____

_____

_____

_____

DATE	MEAL	RECIPE

Recipe Reflections

_____

_____

_____

_____

_____

_____

DATE	MEAL	RECIPE

Recipe Reflections

_____

_____

_____

_____

_____

Made in United States
Troutdale, OR
12/28/2023